MW00907207

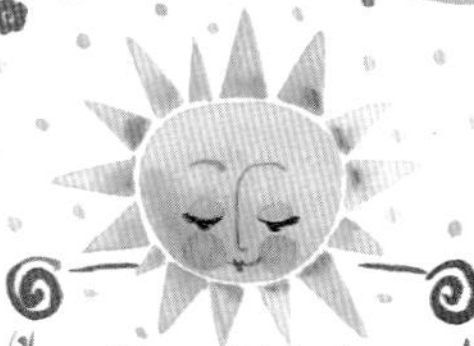

GET WELL SOON

By Nick Beilenson

Illustrated by Kathy Davis
Design by Arlene Greco

PETER PAUPER PRESS, INC.
WHITE PLAINS, NEW YORK

Text copyright © 1997
Peter Pauper Press, Inc.
202 Mamaroneck Avenue
White Plains, NY 10601
Illustrations copyright © 1997
Kathy Davis Designs, Inc.
All Rights Reserved
ISBN 0-88088-825-3
Printed in China
7 6 5 4 3 2 1

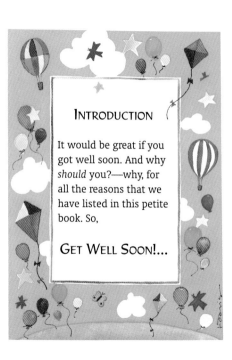

INTRODUCTION

It would be great if you got well soon. And why *should* you?—why, for all the reasons that we have listed in this petite book. So,

GET WELL SOON!...

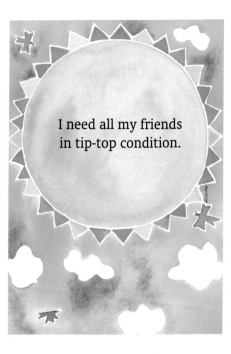

I need all my friends
in tip-top condition.

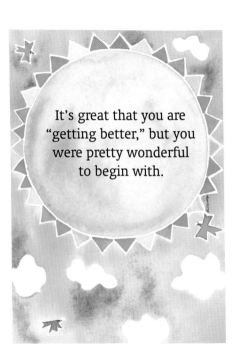

It's great that you are "getting better," but you were pretty wonderful to begin with.

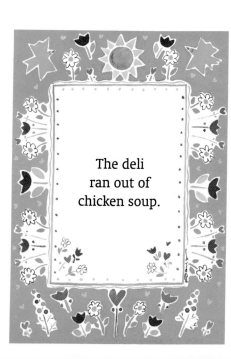

The deli
ran out of
chicken soup.

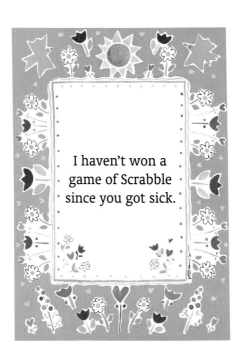

I haven't won a
game of Scrabble
since you got sick.

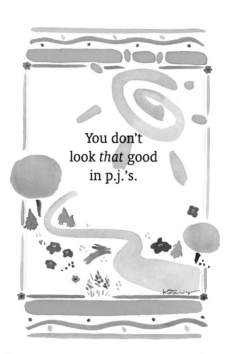

You don't
look *that* good
in p.j.'s.

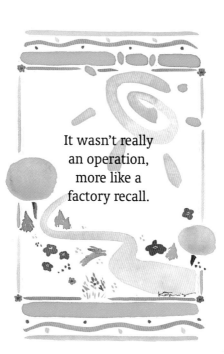

It wasn't really
an operation,
more like a
factory recall.

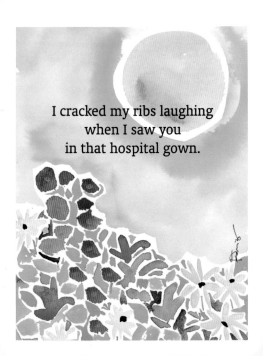

I cracked my ribs laughing
when I saw you
in that hospital gown.

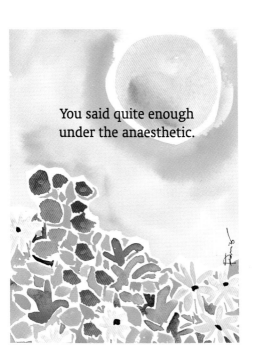

You said quite enough
under the anaesthetic.

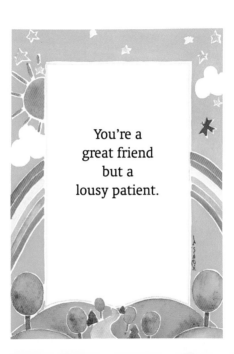

You're a
great friend
but a
lousy patient.

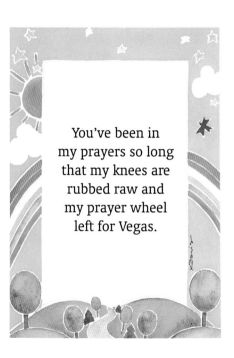

You've been in my prayers so long that my knees are rubbed raw and my prayer wheel left for Vegas.

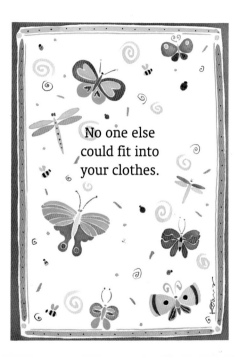

No one else
could fit into
your clothes.

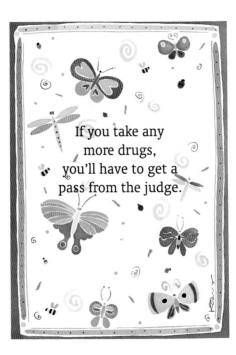

If you take any
more drugs,
you'll have to get a
pass from the judge.

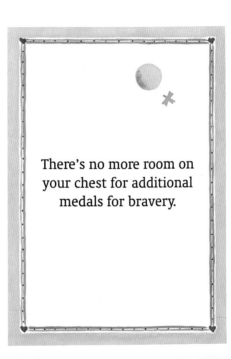

There's no more room on your chest for additional medals for bravery.

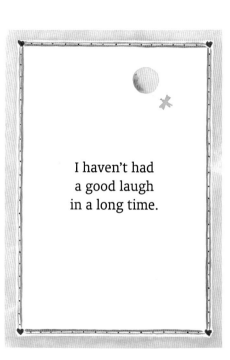

I haven't had
a good laugh
in a long time.

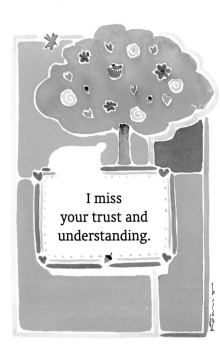

I miss
your trust and
understanding.

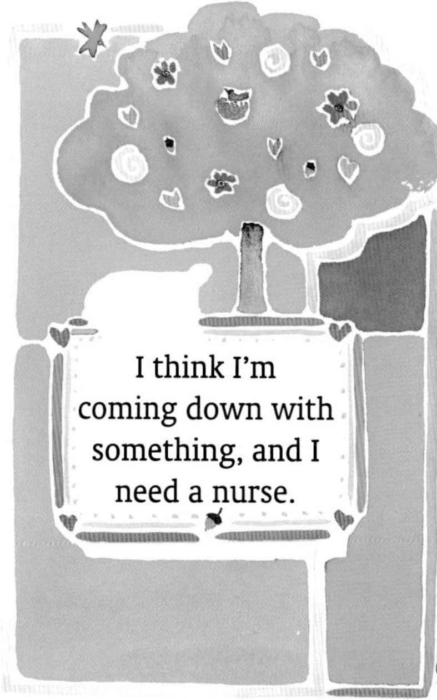
I think I'm
coming down with
something, and I
need a nurse.

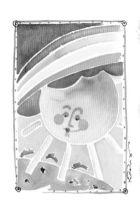

I'm tired of
walking your dog.

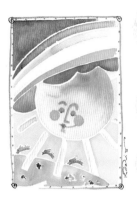

Groaning and moaning
is more effective when
there is a time limit.

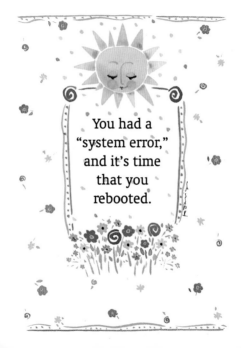

You had a
"system error,"
and it's time
that you
rebooted.

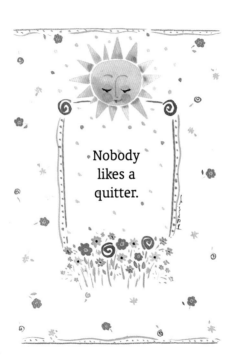

Nobody
likes a
quitter.

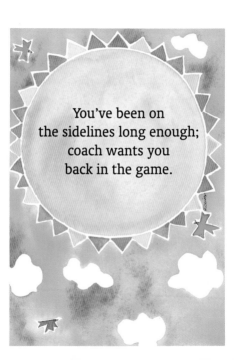

You've been on
the sidelines long enough;
coach wants you
back in the game.

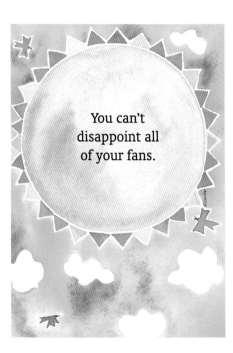

You can't disappoint all of your fans.

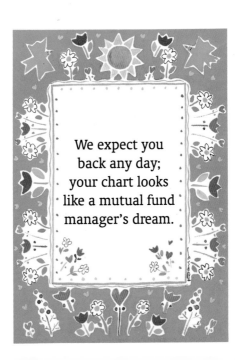

We expect you
back any day;
your chart looks
like a mutual fund
manager's dream.

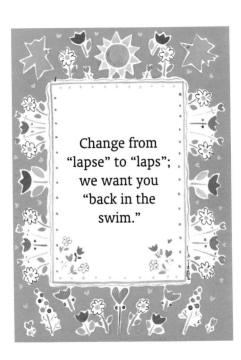

Change from "lapse" to "laps"; we want you "back in the swim."

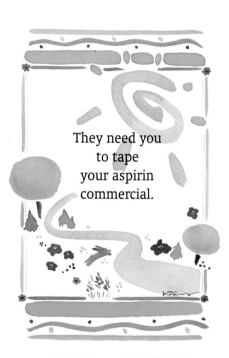

They need you
to tape
your aspirin
commercial.

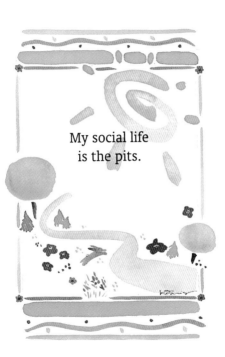

My social life
is the pits.

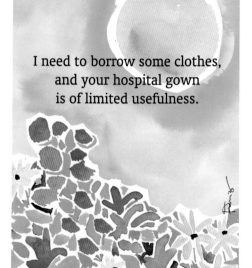

I need to borrow some clothes,
and your hospital gown
is of limited usefulness.

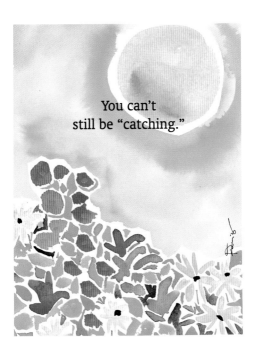

You can't
still be "catching."

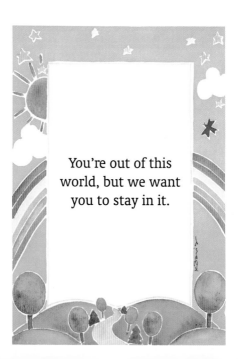

You're out of this world, but we want you to stay in it.

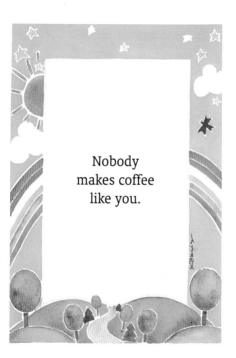

Nobody
makes coffee
like you.

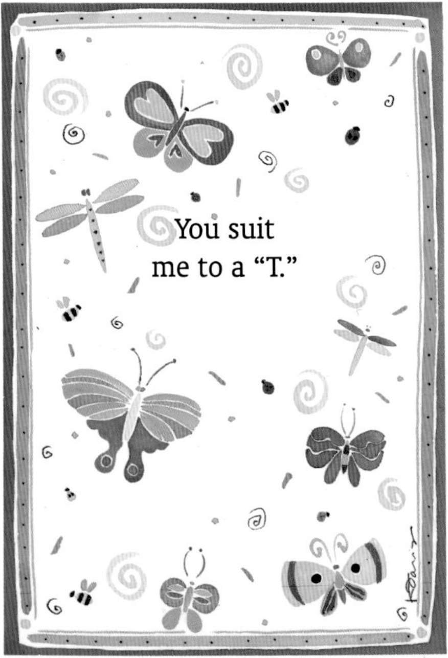
You suit
me to a "T."

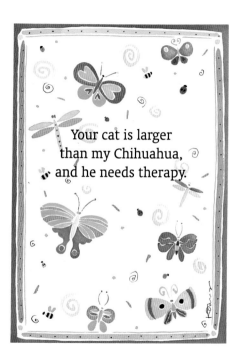

Your cat is larger
than my Chihuahua,
and he needs therapy.

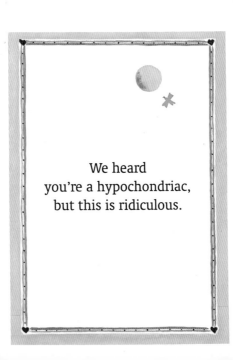

We heard
you're a hypochondriac,
but this is ridiculous.

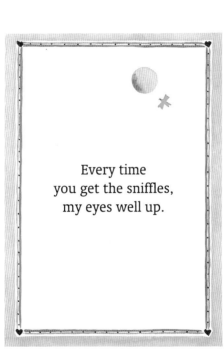

Every time
you get the sniffles,
my eyes well up.

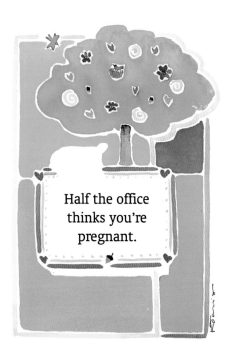

Half the office
thinks you're
pregnant.

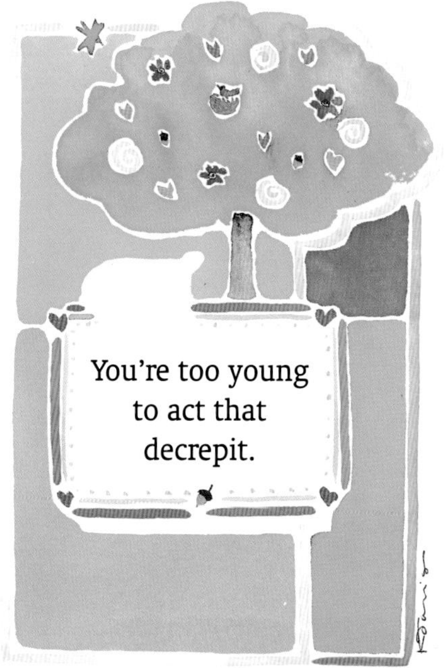
You're too young
to act that
decrepit.

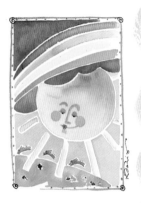

I feel really bad for you,
and I'm getting depressed.

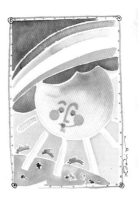

There's a little cloud over my heart,
even on a sunny day.

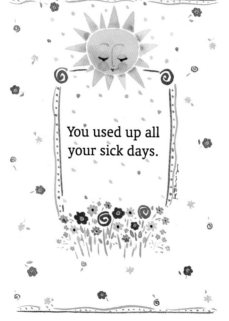

You used up all
your sick days.

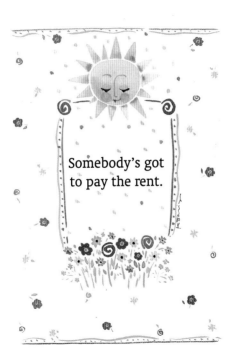

Somebody's got
to pay the rent.

I miss your smile.

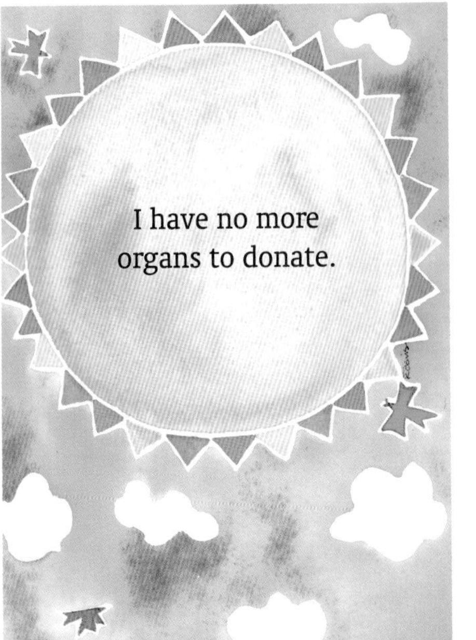
I have no more
organs to donate.

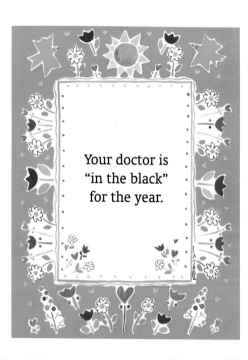

Your doctor is
"in the black"
for the year.

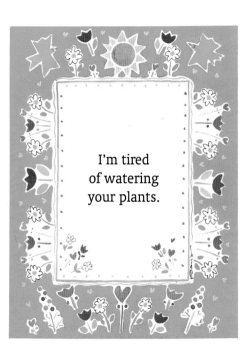

I'm tired
of watering
your plants.

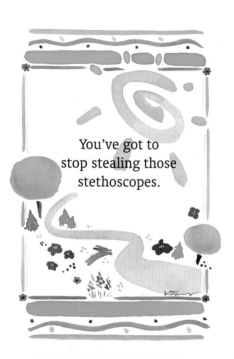

You've got to
stop stealing those
stethoscopes.

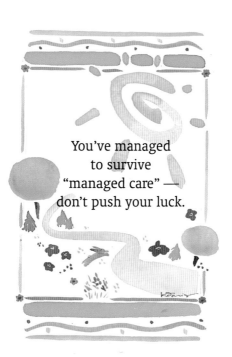

You've managed
to survive
"managed care" —
don't push your luck.

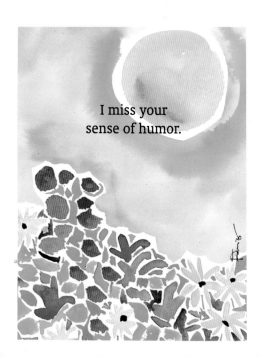

I miss your
sense of humor.

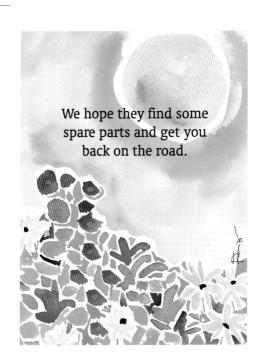

We hope they find some spare parts and get you back on the road.

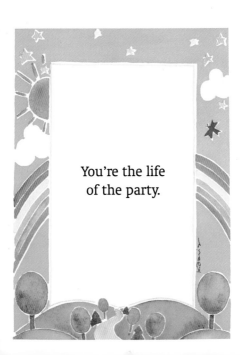

You're the life
of the party.

I need someone
to talk to.

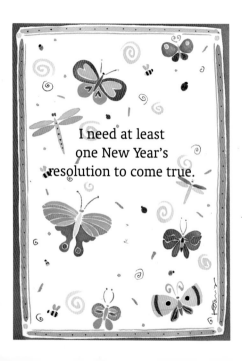

I need at least
one New Year's
resolution to come true.

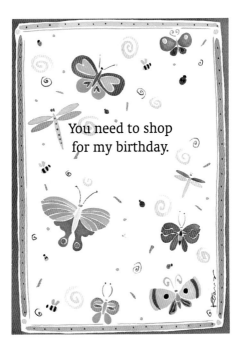

You need to shop
for my birthday.

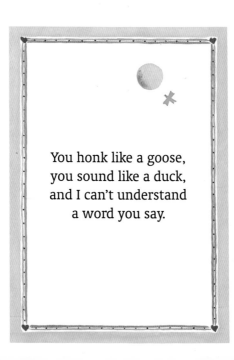

You honk like a goose,
you sound like a duck,
and I can't understand
a word you say.

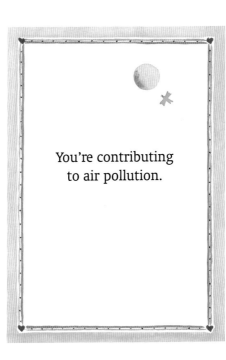

You're contributing
to air pollution.

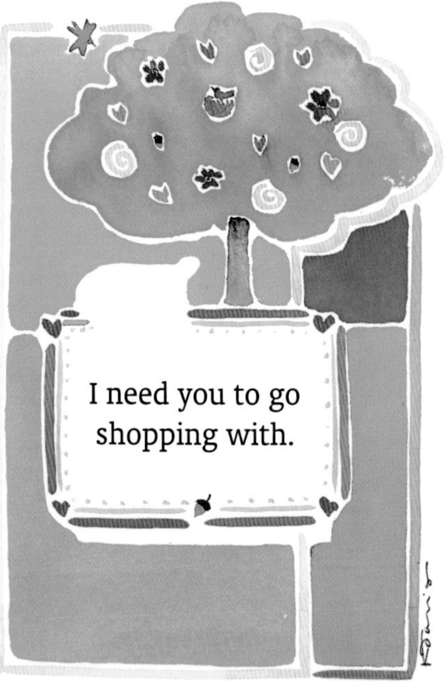
I need you to go shopping with.

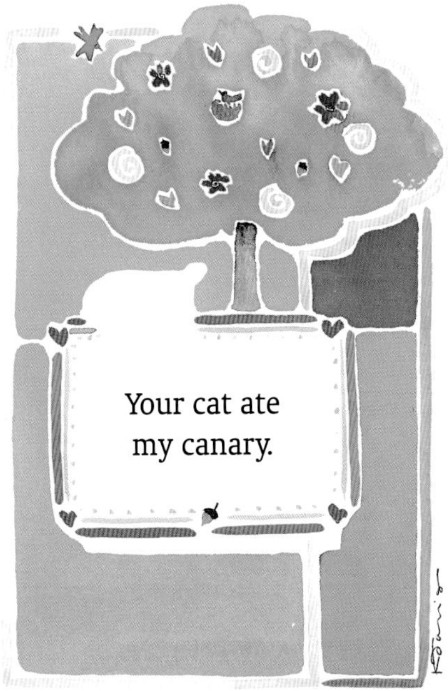
Your cat ate
my canary.

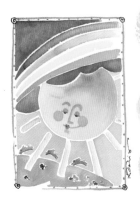

Life just isn't as much fun
without you.

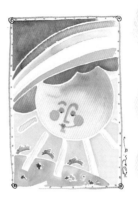

How can we discuss movies
you haven't seen?

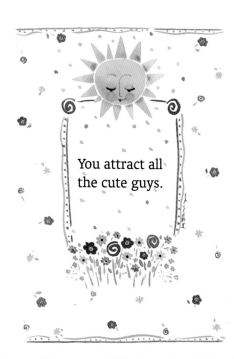

You attract all
the cute guys.

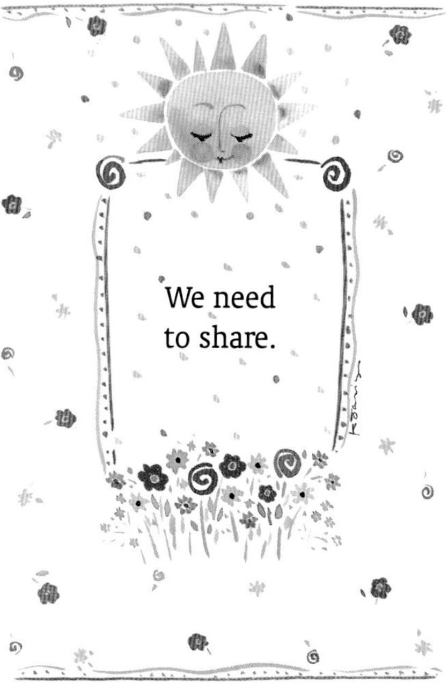

We need
to share.

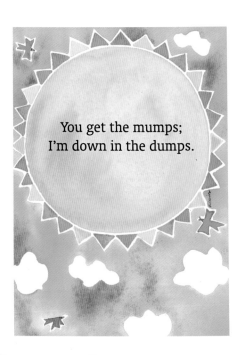

You get the mumps;
I'm down in the dumps.

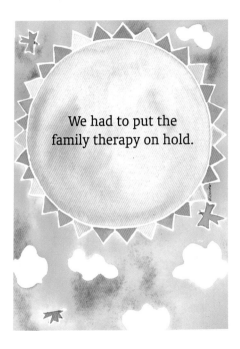

We had to put the family therapy on hold.

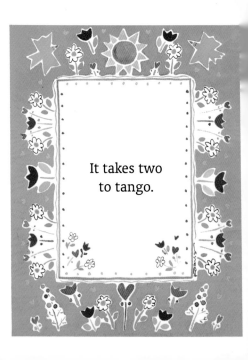

It takes two
to tango.

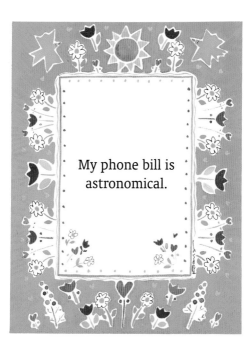

My phone bill is
astronomical.

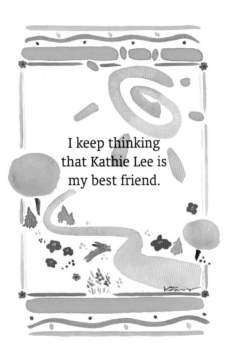

I keep thinking
that Kathie Lee is
my best friend.

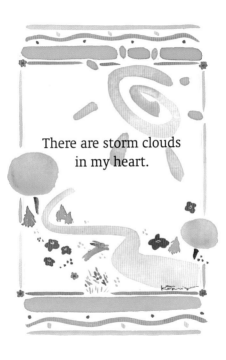

There are storm clouds
in my heart.

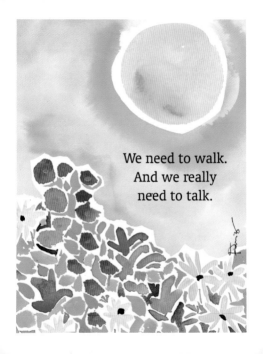

We need to walk.
And we really
need to talk.

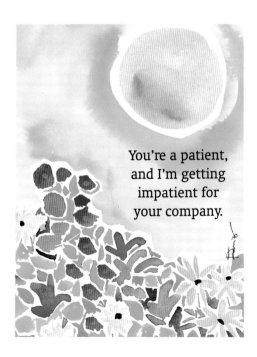

You're a patient,
and I'm getting
impatient for
your company.

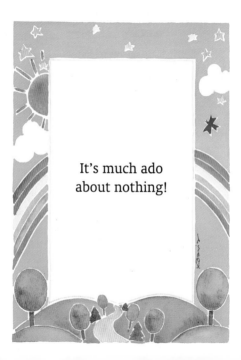

It's much ado
about nothing!

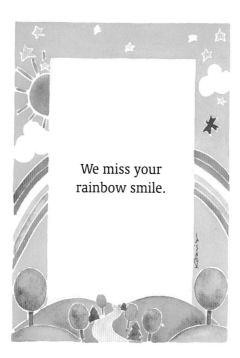

We miss your
rainbow smile.

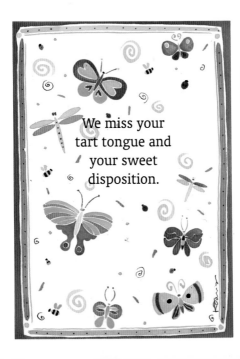

We miss your
tart tongue and
your sweet
disposition.

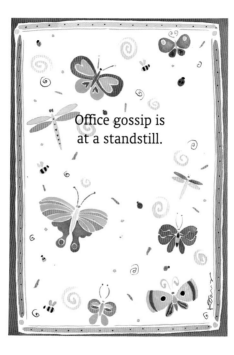

Office gossip is
at a standstill.

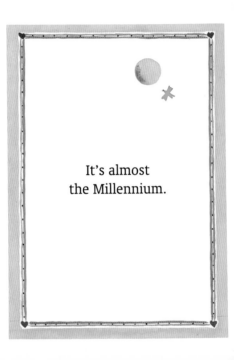

It's almost
the Millennium.

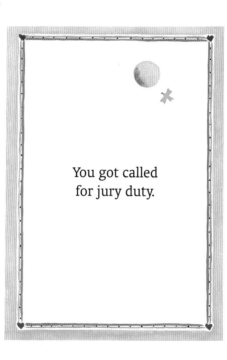

You got called
for jury duty.

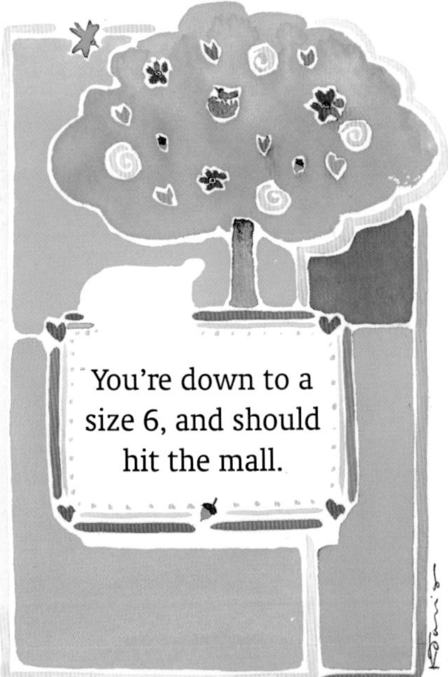
You're down to a
size 6, and should
hit the mall.